Bluewords Greening

Also by Christine Stewart-Nuñez

Untrussed
Keeping Them Alive
Postcard on Parchment

Bluewords Greening

by

Christine Stewart-Nuñez

Terrapin Books

Published by Terrapin Books
4 Midvale Avenue
West Caldwell, New Jersey 07006-8006

ISBN: 978-0-9976666-1-8
LCCN: 2016948352

Visit us at www.terrapinbooks.com

First edition

Cover Art and Design by Megan Nelson

For Holden, my marvel,
Xavier, my miracle,
& Brian, my match

Contents

Epilogue

Prologue

Signing 101

Pay attention, she says, *to relationships—*
how the hands convey meaning in degrees
of proximity to the body. With my index
finger, I point to my chin, tip touching
a dimple I feel but no one sees, and tuck
the rest of my fingers. To sign *miss her,*
I twist my wrist and point to an empty
place, as if the daughter I never birthed
had been there, swaddled, smelling delicate.
If I intend *disappointed,* I hold my hand
in position and think about an attempt
to make a papier-mâché solar system
with my son who has no focus for crafts
or spoken words. *How quickly one sign slides*
into another, a student says. Everyone nods.
To signify *bitter,* my brain need only to dwell
in this hollow, thin-skinned space, my hand
to tighten into a fist.

Book One: Bluewords

Temporary Innocence

Warm water rushes
onto my son's hair;
I massage his curls,
lathering shampoo.
From the side of my
eye, the shower light
looks like a hovering
dove. As suds trickle
over squeezed-shut eyes,
sand drains down pipes
along with stray globs
of sunblock and a splotch
of red paint. I christen
this slippery cherub, he
who shrieks and splashes
as if he'll never feel
the heat of flames,
as if he'll never slip
for a spell, as if he'll
never soar.

Permutations of Light

On the screen, I see how God
has wrapped my son's brain
in light, a glow around gray

folds that house fiber-optic threads
of blood. When lightning storms
here along synaptic clefts, cells

ignite, fire, flare, and surge.
In the nightlight's shine, I've seen
sweat-soaked hair, a twitching cheek,

my son's rigid body. The time
I held him in a highway's ditch—
brown and stiff autumn grasses

poking out of snow—his legs
were limp, the wells of his eyes fixed
heavenward as if in supplication.

Caressing his perfect skin, I whispered,
You'll be fine in a minute, you'll be fine
until my mantra persuaded even

the blue sky, its sunlight folding
into April's awakening fields. Light
held me when his jaw locked—vomit

forced through his nose, and it steadied
me when we spent three silent hours
in the emergency room. There's the light

in his eyes when he cracks a joke
and the way his words spark like fireflies
at dusk. That night when he stepped out

of the hospital, he looked into the sky,
spied the waxing moon, and yelled,
Yahoooooo!

Naming

I named my child Holden not
after a book character
or a soap opera hunk,
but because Holden sounds
solid and stable, because it
means calm and gracious—good
attributes for a man—
and because it stems from
a hollow in the valley
which summons memories
of camping between forested hills
along the Mississippi, of nights
staring into bonfires and stargazing
believing God was there—Infinity
in constellations and flames.

It wasn't until Holden
was four years old that I typed
seizure disorder into a search engine
for the one-thousandth time
and was struck by meaning.
"Epilepsy: from Greek
leps-, stem
of lambanein—
to take
hold of."

Solving for Epilepsy

In the hospital, my son sleeps,
his body's shape a curved
petal, a question mark. The MRI
shows an illuminated walnut,
gray-white matter without blight.

A yellow-green sky precedes
evening tornadoes; fever
forewarns seizures. I kiss-check
his forehead for heat each minute.

Distinguish a daydream
from a quick spell: snow
falls; falling snow. I pull
his ear to gauge reaction.
Stop it, Mom, he says.

I type "spring buds, ruby
balloons" as he catches a dust
speck with his gaze. Purple
hydrangea: his brain balanced
upon its stem, blooming.

A fuzzy mirror, he says,
crumpling. Through
this fog, does he see
my mouth move, hear
the ping of counted seconds
on the roof of his skull?

A medieval saint suggests a cure:
cake of mole blood, duck beak,
goose feet, wheat flour. He pops
six pills in the morning, nine at
night. *Learn to hunt,* I vow.

Pick a Play

One doctor describes the neurons
in my son's brain as fans
in a stadium who, when cheerleaders
start The Wave, stand and throw
their arms in the air regardless
of hand-held hotdogs and Cokes.
In a minute or two, the cells
have their butts back in the seats
and my son squeezes my elbow.

Sometimes, he's in the game
but runs a silent play: the coin
revolves mid-air, fumbled pigskin
suspended before it hits the ground,
a split-second frame of cleat-meets-ball.
Will he remember the field where
we kicked and caught in a blizzard
of cottonwood seeds, tufts floating by
at our every turn? Will he even recall
the picnic of bubbles, glassy spheres
sailing between us as we twirled,
plastic wands in our hands?

The clock ticks in his brain's
continuous game. Men crash
into other men, smack helmets.
The occasional crunch
of tendon or bone. I don't care
if a quarter ends with a touchdown
or without a score as long
as clusters of neurons stand separately
to cheer, one fan zipping a sweater,
another sipping a beer.

Portraits Before Epileptic Aphasia

1.

After Holden's international flight
touches down in Kraków, after he refuses
bread despite hunger, and after he strips
down to big-boy shorts white and tight
around his waist, he flits from pillow
to pillow. He lifts his orange cast, arm
broken by a jump from a slide, and puffs
out his chest. It's midnight. He kicks
his pajamas and tumbles after them, giggling.
I gather him up. His back arcs, body
turning out toward the window thrown
open to the spring night. My hold
around his waist tightens. I sing
until his wings surrender.

2.

Imagination and reality collapse:
shoulders flush with the wall, Holden
listens for pirates. The brown irises
of his eyes sparkle as he clanks down
the hotel's halls in sailor boots: *Shhhh...*
they're following me, he says. After seeing
fire-breathing dragon statues, castles
lined with armor-clad knights, and crystal-
coated caves, anything's possible. He spies
the Jolly Roger and claims the treasure
chest with his heel. In books, his shadow
could peel itself off the wall and search
for more gold. For now he purses his full
lips and thinks the shadows alive.

3.

I can't explain Auschwitz-Birkenau
to Holden, so he doesn't go. I can't
explain piles of children's school shoes,

galoshes, Dutch clogs; stacks of baskets
and suitcases with numbers chalked in white;
mounds of human hair and textiles made
from it. Ash, fat, bones used for *things*.
Shafts of light show where Nazis dropped
Zyklon B. For *efficiency, experiments.*

What would Holden think of my weeping
as I imagine mothers hugging their children
as gas infused the air? Behind a fence, I glimpse
a cottage and imagine a garden—lilies, lilacs,
lettuce, dill—and the commandant's children
romping around in the clothes of the dead.

4.

We take refuge from rain in a café
and order szarlotka—apples encased
in a buttery-sweet crust; tiramisu—
tiers of mascarpone, lady-fingers,
and liqueur-infused cocoa; dark
chocolate cake—bitterness countered
with sugar and cream; crepes—disks
drizzled with orange sauce. All delightful.
But Holden's hot cocoa alters
expectations: layers of steamed milk,
melted chocolate, whipped cream.
If only these reversals—dessert as
dinner, layered hot chocolate, not mixed—
could sweeten those to come. I spoon
riches onto Holden's ready tongue.

5.

Just after sunset, we find the right
platform, proper train, assigned car,
correct couchette. Holden squawks
at the bunk's tight fit; I insist we share,
spooning in a nest of sweatshirts.
A train, a train, we'll sleep on a train,
he says. So different than his toy's

wooden tracks. *Listen for the whistle,*
I whisper. The train picks up speed.
Remember this, I think. Rolling through
the Polish countryside, the breeze
from the open window kisses his hair.

6.

We walk Prague's streets, serpentine
paths on the map. Right angles morph
into loops and curve into splashes
of green, blue, gray—the same as grassy
parks, pastel buildings, steel-hued clouds.
Near a playground, public art: a faceless
human positioned on elbows and knees,
a huge skull bowing its back. Holden tiptoes
around *Parable of a Skull* without placing
his arm inside the empty eye socket
or sliding his hand down the cold thigh
yet scrutinizes it. I open my mouth, words
two-dimensional like our map's key.
He turns and solves the moment:
Why's he crawling? Babies crawl.

7.

At the Wallenstein Gardens,
Holden chases white peacocks
through hedges, branches scratching
his legs. At a dead-end in the maze,
he gets close; he digs into his pocket
for a biscuit. The bird steps, chest
puffed, and turns his crowned head.
Their eyes lock. Lunge, snap.
An empty hand. I fear sharp beak
near child skin, and yet the fan
of white eyes consumes me. I hold
a dropped feather against my chest
and hope, even as its colors shift
in the light, that they never change.

8.

Holden grasps the vintage camera
to steady it. Into the viewfinder
he presses his eye, and his uncle guides:
You can change what you see: fuzzy
or close up? Someday, Holden may
manipulate focus and scope, skew
his view, warp beauty, find an angle
of light in a somber shot. On this trip,
new frames shape his point of view:
zigzagging through vineyards, scaling castle
steps, studying a hornless rhino, finding
chocolate ladybugs on hotel pillows.
Plucked out of the buzz of regular life,
I observe him zooming on a train toward
the Bavarian Film Studios, documenting
his life with images, without words.

Buffaloed

Before Holden's five-year-old brain
changed; before the slow-wave-and-spikes
during sleep eroded concentration;
before his deep-brown eyes glazed over
with confusion; before he tossed
a handful of pills across the kitchen;
before he squeezed tears away with fists;
before he threw himself in the snow
to protest a scheduled blood draw;
before he spit anger from his mouth;
before words got lost between mind
and tongue,
              he told me one morning:
I dreamed a buffalo kissed me on the forehead.

Epiphany

It happens like this: information accumulates
like a slow rain, scattered drops taking hours
to equal a quarter inch. Your preschooler turns away
from *Want ice cream?* without an answer. He mimics
dialogue from *Monsters Inc.* and recites *Yoshi's Feast*
after breakfast, in the car, as he falls asleep.
Blank stares add up; you blink concerns away.
You invent reasons: medication, exhaustion, like
his father, a phase. Glacial, understanding's time;
it arrives the afternoon he drops a glass. Shards slide
across the kitchen floor. He plunges his whole self
toward the sparkly ice, your body a wedge
between his screams and the glass he intends to eat.
No words you speak—*it's dangerous, calm down,
we'll get another*—quell his desperation. As you sweep
up the mess into a skillet with bare hands, he climbs
over your back. Realization crystallizes—face it! face it!—
something's just not right.

Elusive Diagnosis

Saturated with sleeplessness, a drug-induced
haze, Holden stares at Ireland's misted fields.
Seizures spike in his brain each minute he sleeps

while a question bombards mine: how does
154 days of Valium help? Irish air tastes
of too much nectar and honey, fruit near rot,

yet May's viridian won't turn its hip
into yellow until autumn. The neurologist
prescribed but didn't name the what and why

and how. What happens beyond two minds
so thoroughly soaked, so thoroughly charged
with not knowing? Such humidity. Trees along

the highway steam. Meadows, so purely green,
hurt my eyes. The sheep we count in sleep
are fenced by stone hedges. The car stops.

We stroll inside a ruined chapel amid its
congregation of grass. A black lamb
beyond the gate bleats: *Wring out the wet*

wool over your eyes. Seaside, when you sought
shells but found sharp rocks, then—at least—
you found an answer.

Art of the Body

after Aquaform by Pauline Aitken

I see art in the body and the body in art
no matter where I look on this wall:
in canvases, in my son's darting shadow.

Aquaform, with its nucleus at the heart,
membranes and organelles I'll call
these shapes, and I'll make this a window

to consider seizures, how they part
neurons and words, how they stall
my son's learning. Mine feels shallow:

on a gallery walk, thoughts start.
I focus first, then fall
into paint, into cells, into sorrow.

Into paint, into cells, into sorrow
I focus first, then fall.
On a gallery walk, my thoughts start—

my son's learning. Mine feels shallow.
Neurons and words—how they stall
to consider seizures, how they part

these images and make this a window.
Membranes and organelles I'll call
Aquaform, with its nucleus at the heart.

In canvases, in my son's darting shadow,
no matter where I look on this wall,
I see art in the body and the body in art.

Lexicon for Landau-Kleffner Syndrome

sei*zure

To confiscate my son's concentration
and consciousness. To arrest. He points,
Fuzzy mirror! steps backward, and folds
his legs like a colt. *Happy birthday to you,
happy birthday*—a breathy version of the song
we'd sung earlier to his grandmother.
For 118 seconds, his hand squeezes
and squeezes until his brain releases him.

a*no*mi*a

To have trouble finding the correct word.
We weave through a throng of blue-and-yellow-
clad fans bottlenecked at the street's end,
and we step aside when the band saunters by
with trombones slung over their shoulders.
The homecoming parade's dispersing. My kid
grasps his bag of Bubblegum, Pixie Sticks,
and Tootsie Rolls thrown from the floats:
That was a great candy store, Mom!

To substitute correct names of words.
He watches a prairie landscape video,
wind howling, and says: *I hear the dust.*

e*cho*la*li*a

To imitate sounds without expressive awareness,
as if planning a proposal, untangling meaning,
memorizing lines, studying for an exam. No.
No deliberateness—a record skipping, skipping:

               I want
                       to play
                               mini-ninjas. I want to play
                                       mini-ninjas. I want
                       to play mini-ninjas. Mini-ninjas.
                               Mini-ninjas. I want
                                   to play
               mini
                                       ninjas.
                       Mini-ninjas? Mini-ninjas?
               I want
                       to
                               play
                                       mini-ninjas.

ne*ol*o*gi*sms

To coin new words. He pauses before
baskets of peppers in the produce aisle—
yellow-green Anaheims, full-pocketed
poblanos, comma-thin Thais, Fresno reds,
holy jalapeños, orange Scotch bonnets:
Look! Hotchiladas!

A coined phrase based on visual evidence.
The meal: bowl of rice, stir-fry shrimp,
pineapple, mushrooms, soy sauce, and Sriracha—
rooster emblazoned on the bottle in white.
In his words, *Cockadoodle spicy!*

re*cep*tive lang*uage loss

Language comprehension deficit. The game
of broken telephone, grapevine, whisper down
the lane, pass the message—storming synapses

scatter meaning, words enter his ear and evaporate
again and again, over and over:

  Mom?!
    Right here.
  Nothing.
    Okay.
  Sorry!
    No worries.
  You're welcome.

As if swabs of damp cotton in his ears.
Does he hear me like the adults in *Peanuts*
cartoons: *Whaa, whaa whaa, whaaaaa?*
I test what's getting through:

  Do you want chocolate?
    No.
  A movie?
    No.
  A kitten?
    No.
  Trip to Disney World?
    I don't want to talk about it.

ex*pres*sive lang*uage loss

The inability to express one's self.
A summer day he stops riding his bike
and leans on the left side, training wheels
about to give. I start:

  We have to go home.
    NO!
  Come on. We have to go this way.
    No, no, no!
  Come on, let's go.
    Nooooooooooo.
  Holden, we have to GO. We can't stand here. You
    almost got hit by a car.

We have to take the sidewalk. He hangs his head and
   cries. I rub his back.
*Come on, sweetheart. We have to go. Do you want me to
   carry you?*
   Noooooooooo.
Do you want Mom to help?
   NO!!!!!
What's the matter? Huh? What's the matter?
   Inaudible whine. *It's.... stuck.*
What? Your handle bar? Let me fix it. See? Don't lean.
   Thank you.

He rides on the sidewalk until home.

Kindling

In neurology, the tendency of some regions of the brain to react to repeated low-level bioelectrical stimulation by progressively boosting synaptic discharges, thereby lowering seizure thresholds.

Minutes slip into an abyss
when neuron activity shifts.
He steps out wet with piss.
Minutes slip into an abyss
as messages surge; they miss
or meet along axonic rifts.
Minutes slip—an abyss
of neuron activity shifts.

A seizure pattern—cells adapt;
neurons, like dry twigs, combust
and flames spread, paths remapped.
A seizure pattern. Cells adapt
and singe words, language capped.
How much damage from just
a seizure pattern? Cells adapt:
neurons, like dry twigs, combust.

What happens to a brain
burning for years and years?
Will flames make its impact plain?
What happens to a brain
smoldering with a chain
of seizures if no cure appears?
What happens to a brain
burning? Fears and fears.

Learn by Doing

Let's do fireworks! my six-year-old shouts,
pushing a sparkler box into my hand.
He presses one into a flame, and it sprouts

sparks. Fingers on the wire, he commands
the fire, staring into the star's center.
Pushing a sparkler box into my hand,

my kid's ideas quicken. His friends stir
the air, wands writing. Not my son's
fire-stick. Staring into the star's center,

he raises the orb, eye-level, and jettisons
fear. Near his cheek, sparks leap
into air. Wands write, but not my son's.

If I let him hold a fistful, he'd creep
closer to the bursts, lips pursed.
No fear. Near his cheek, sparks leap

to graze his skin. He's still curious.
More fireworks! my six-year-old shouts.
Closer to the burst, lips pursed,
he presses the flame; fascination sprouts.

Aphasia Ironies

The professor's son
sighs, sulks, and bolts when "school" slips
through his locked mind's maze.

The writer's son won't
grasp wood; penciled letters melt
into squiggled strings.

The poet's son lost
language, his seizure-stabbed brain
a sieve oozing words.

Thirteen Ways of Understanding Blueword

Blueword: any given word spoken by someone with aphasia

1.
Among one million combinations
the only uttered thing
was the syllable of a blueword.

2.
The boy is eternally present
like a mouth
speaking blueword, blueword, blueword.

3.
The blueword disappeared on the cusp of a dream.
It was one memory lost in a seizing brain.

4.
A boy and a thought
sync up.
A boy and a thought and a blueword
sync up.

5.
I do not know which to prefer,
My nerves are gone,
or *Nerf gun? Nerf gun? I want a Nerf gun,*
the blueword appearing
or just leaving.

6.
Brain waves filled the paper
with abnormal data,
the outline of bluewords
scribbled up and down.
A symptom
translated when he writes,
hand revealing all.

7.

O grown ups in my life,
why do you imagine me a comedian?

Do you not hear the bluewords
shift as you sleep? You're adults;
adults are chameleons.

8.

Blue blue blue
Blue world, blue wood
Blue bird, word, blue

WORD, blueword

9.

When a blueword softened
into a pool of silence, it smudged
the edge of understanding.

10.

At the sound of a string of bluewords
arriving in syntactical precision,
even the speech pathologist
would applaud wildly.

11.

He listens for his past
before a computer screen.
Once, longing piqued him
in that he remembered a time
without a blueword.

12.

Summer rain shakes the linden tree's leaves.
The blueword must be fluttering.

13.
It was midnight all morning.
Seizures were spiking
and they were going to spike.
The blueword lodged
in the back of his throat.

Ode to Echolalia

O, Chatter! *Who? Who? Don't know!*
He giggles and mouths the window.

Sunshine, lollipops, ever'thing he sings
for me to puzzle out. He brings

lines of lyrics, phrases from TV;
these word-rhythms make a spree

of sound from his jubilant tongue. *Juice!*
I think he's put his thirst to use,

but he pushes the glass away.
O, Chatter! *Go, go, go, now stay—*

this book bit cuts the silence
of his fog-dimmed brain. Shyness

it's not, the sullen spells of quiet.
So come, Chatter, come riot

of repetitive sound. You're
my money maker and marrow builder,

my music and muse mover, my solace
that syllables slide through *his* lips

into *my* ear. You're his grasp,
his tether, his thought on the cusp

of expression even though
his mind is working, working slow.

O Echolalia! Remind me
of your virtues when occasionally

his cheeks quiver and mouth twitches—
frustration on his face as he pitches

puffs of air instead of words—
breaking, for a moment, my heart.

Lessons in Context

No means
maybe. No
means *you're*
annoying me
with sounds,
can't you see
this game
right here?,
your questions
hurt my ears.
No means
yes, if you
ask again in
five minutes.
No means
I see your
moving lips,
and so? No
means *no.*
Sometimes.
No means
I hate that
t-shirt, I'm
sick of swallowing
chalk, that kid
over there
smells like pee.
No means *I'm*
thinking; persuade me
with marshmallows.
No means *sometimes,*
I enjoy pissing you off.
No means
you're clueless.
You don't know

what this is like;
here, I'll throw
myself on the ground
screaming and weeping
to give you
a little taste.

Mistakes in Museums

For the art museum's reception, I dress
my infant in his best clothes, cotton
sleeper soft against olive-toned skin.
The air is cool. I cover all exposed skin,
a few curls of brown hair I failed to dress
peeking out from the cap of blue cotton.
Perhaps it's more than his cotton
clothing that compels her, but a stranger skins
our pleasure: *He looks like Taliban in that dress.*
I don't dress her down or cotton to; I thicken my skin.

At the children's museum, my second-grade son
and I build walls with blue foam cubes. A boy
joins us. Holden's silence doesn't bother him.
Did you meet Holden at school? I ask him.
Yes, this younger child says. *I know your son,
he's different.* He brings a block to my boy,
then places it on Holden's. *He's a boy
like me*, he says. I wonder about him—
what he's been told about my son.
Your son is a boy, but is he human? He points to him.

Literacy

Inside GameStop, I find Holden kneeling
in front of Xbox, Wii, Nintendo, PlayStation,
a display of plastic boxes arranged on shelves.

Screens again, I sigh. Plants shooting peas
and slogging zombies, fat red birds launched
at green pigs, jigsaws, a library of Dr. Seuss,

episodes of Word Girl defending cartoon land
against Lady Redundant Woman—his iPad
the visual center of his word-shifting world.

He studies the spines, lifts his hand, extends
his fingers, and pulls one game off. *Sonic*, he says,
opening it, *Sonic the Hedgehog*. He points to letters

on the inner pocket: *Sonic the Hedgehog. I know
this game.* This will be his only utterance for hours.
As he snaps the plastic cover closed and slides

it back, a memory emerges: my hand easing
On the Banks of Plum Creek next to the other
Little House books, the scent of paperbacks
and pencil shavings, dust swirling in the air.

Boy at Rest

after Julie Zick's *Girl at Rest*

> *While sleeping, the child vanishes from his life.*
> —Carolyn Forché, *The Angel of History*

In *Girl at Rest*, I saw only a hazy
silhouette of a child's body—the navy
blue frame of her arms, head,

and a bit of torso. And I read
the artist's choice of ochre and light
gray—shades shifting only slightly—

to convey background and skin
with wonder: the colors nearly vanish
the child. When I study my son

asleep, it's in full dimension:
eyelids threaded with a blue vein,
a freckle emerging on the outline

of his lip. There's no facial stress,
but I don't need to guess:
rest is an illusion, not a feature

of a brain besot by seizures.
By day, they complicate the spelling
of C-A-T, blur the way sounds, rolling

into each other, infuse meaning.
When sound does get through the screen
of spells, a word may fail to find its place

on his tongue. The seizures also erase
memories of lunchtime pizza, gym-class
tag, the answer to *What's your last*

name? the need to look both ways before
crossing the parking lot outside the store.
On the monitor, I hear him speak,

a midnight phrase thrown from deep sleep,
and I wonder what words emerge
(despite the seizure's surge)

from the visual play of his dreams.
What world does he vanish to? It seems
impossible to draw in ink or words

more than a sleeping child's curves
and angles. When I tiptoe into his room
to re-tuck his blanket, I'll only assume

that wherever he's at,
                              he'll come back.

Lithography

On the stone of my body, I drew you
indelible, unique—cliché yet true—
and the world's ink rolled over us.
Fusions. Variations. You repelled
my blonde hair, fair skin, and blue
eyes—our shared nose less obvious.

On the stone of my body, I drew you
yet this art process I've borrowed is a clue
to why you are you. Acid's dangerous
but it etches beauty. Son, you resist
my moves, my words, but in my view
we're art *because* of what life puts us through.

Mutations

after Lynda Benglis's *Los Angeles 1984 Olympic Games*

Black, red, yellow and blue rings
overlap in this print's center, morph
into strings of cells, folded membranes
and organelles floating in a wash
of green, a sweep of yellow. Mutant
cells, I think, mutants like the tribe
of blue-eyeds begun in an ancestor
of mine 10,000 years ago. I missed
expressing other mistakes—red hair
and freckles. Sixty or so errors spring up
in anyone's genetic code; my son's
de novo mutation, GRIN2A, the cause
of word-erosion. Like these circle-cells
splitting, my genes and his father's tangled
and tore away imperfectly. And yet.
Mitochondrial Eve—mutant child—
helped bring humans back from the brink
of extinction; did she marvel at her difference?
Perhaps a life lived longer? Or stronger?
Will we ever see GRIN2A as a beautiful
mistake? My son on the cusp of a shift
in *Homo sapiens*, one where speech
succumbs to images, a grand reveal
we're now too shortsighted to see.

Viriditas

This green lives in fire, shimmers in water, moistens stone...
—Heinrich Schipperges, writing of Hildegard's "greening"

In frame after frame, Holden photographed
greenness: pine needles, a trellis of vines, oak
leaves, lawn. The entire frame of variegated
hostas is filled with unfurling flags of summer,
some with lime centers outlined in chartreuse,
others green as grass. The leftmost leaf lolls
like a tongue, the rest curved with curled tips.
He looks so closely, as if ready to lick
the leaf, and why not? When we weeded
the herb garden, we pinched off new dill, broke
off stems of parsley, tasted ribbons of chives.
With each nibbled sprout of cilantro, his eyes
brightened, each burst of flavor settling,
rain-ripened and raw, in his throat.

Hildegard said the soul is like sap, a body-syrup,
a greening energy. Like her, I believe meaning
quickens from within, sometimes slow
as it does in a womb and a seed, sometimes
explosive as it does from a host of ginger
in the mouth and a brain beset with seizures.
Holden's photo that won the art competition:
a green cactus with spines that could prick
a finger and pin a tongue, and yet the image
invites us: taste life with succulent eyes.

Interlude

Metaphysics & Semiotics

1.

Before we sense, we *apprehend*
with our souls, wrote Hildegard.
At three years old, she saw
a *dazzling light*; at five, predicted
an unborn calf's color correctly.
At three years old, my son pointed
to my belly: *Baby in there.* He *knew*
even though I'd just found out.
At six, Holden saw a fuzzy mirror
and stepped back into a seizure
while 1500 miles away, twenty
first-graders were shot in school.
Whose knowledge exhausts
the possibilities of perception?
One man without eyes sees
volume, distance, and shape via
echoes of his clicking tongue.

2.

When Holden's aphasia wanes,
he says *snack booth* for vending
machine, *Lunchable food aisle* instead
of grocery store. Hildegard coined
over 1,000 nouns where words
in German and Latin existed.
Before words, we think in *images,*
odors, flavors, said a linguist;
during the years language left,
Holden thought in images processed
in a healthy part of his brain.
Now when my son speaks, his is not
a quirky kid's cuteness, nor a poet's
desire for heightened diction, nor
a saint's reach for the power of naming.
With pinkie and index fingers up

and thumb out, I push the sign
for love into his line of vision.
I love you, too, he says, then extends
meaning by curling his fingers
around mine and squeezing.

It's "The Journey"

after *Sojourner* by Diana Behl

I'm tempted to clip lines, snip apart
a surface of syntax, toss up a strip
of sky-surfing letters, puzzle word-petals
into corollas. In Behl's print, her petals
of pink paper were never whole. My strip
of words, turning in air, will part
ways, too, transformed. Each sashimi strip
and hair ribbon, all gladiola petals
and beetle wings, will become a part of a new part:
gladwings, hairstrip, bugpetals.

Variables Intrinsic to Printmaking, to Procreation

*Printmaking is an indirect means of creating art by
transferring an image or design by contact with a matrix
such as a block, plate, stone, or screen.*

artist's proof
      portraits of
            roast profit
                 stair fort
premium print
      trimmer pin up
            immune trip
                 item ruin
my son, my a/p
      spy any mom
            pansy, O my!
                 May posy
impressions
      permissions
            promise in
                 imposer
after him
      frame hit
            Father I
                 fear it
flawed, just
      fluted jaws
            just awful
                 deaf lust
as iterations
      aortae insist
            to a inertia
                 I atone air
with each
      ache with
            what ice
                 a white

night's press.
    press things.
        then sprigs.
            the spring.

Book Two: Greening

Conjuring Practice

after *Aerial Crop Rows* by Denise DuBroy

Maize, lime, cherry—the artist planted
colors, bright furrows on the canvas,
crop rows as straight as those I drift
past as waves of weather drift
over my car, snowflakes planted
into my windshield, a white canvas
of sky pressing down. If I canvass
fields for spirals and whorls in drifts—
signatures of wind, paw and plant—
will I find a planted canvas in the drifts?

That Sticky Tango

of bodies, hips
gripped and lips
locked—swing!
it's that skin-to-skin,
all for the win, gin-
enhanced dance
between us

that sticky tango
of sound—*sssss*,
shush, gasp
and whisper,
mmmms end (we
think) with sweaty
hands clutched, my
cheek to your chest

that sticky tango
of sperm, *salida
simple*—a promenade
in the sap of you
until one penetrates
(world within world)
my spinning egg

that sticky tango—
a tangle of genes
enganche, protein
leg wrapped by
protein leg then
split—bit of
you, bit of me
fusing (unknown
to us) and building
a separate he/she.

The Cosmic Tree at Conception

All living creatures are...sparks from the radiation of
God's brilliance.
        —Hildegard of Bingen

As I salute
the sun, my arm
reaches, wrist
arcing like
a chokecherry
branch. Sway,
flex, reach for
faraway stars.
My body's
greening, line
between heaven
and earth
dissolved.
A melody
murmurs, unlocks
muscles along
my spine.
As if spun
gold, my womb
shines; inside,
a spark glows
and a silver
filament
threads
the lining.
Breathe.
I and not I
am the center
of this world.

Framing Loss

On New Year's it attached.
By March—nose fully formed—
it disappeared as before, clots
of tissue floating in the toilet
like some exotic lily. A garden
grew on my table: ruffled
daffodils, yellow crocus, tight
buds of tulips cut too soon.
If sorrow yields sacred ground,
my body blooms hosannas.
No cathedral of cells or city
of organs fills my core, only
the sound of time: wind
humming across fields.
As I once knew budding life,
I feel its vibration seconds before
gusts shake ash tree leaves.
In January, snowflakes filled
the countryside. Now, in cold
ditches and pockets of unbroken
earth—where we expect nothing—
the lavender pasque flower
pushes through spring's snow.

Hildegard's Theories Explain My Miscarriage

I don't heat
slow and steady.
Flame-flung on
the threshing-floor,
my flesh, a lyre,
sings fire.
My beloved's
fingers fan open
envelopes
of skin; air
strokes chords
of tendon, plucks
nerves. Vibrations
spread. Want
harnesses want,
a convection
between bodies.

A hot gust
lines my lips
with dirt. From this
love's tempest,
I take sickness.
The wind feeds
an aerial fire,
dries up life
and bleeds out
my composition.

The nun advised
glow; I hold
my cold skin
and smolder.

How Such Constraints Unbind

And there is pansies. That's for thoughts.
        —Ophelia in *Hamlet*

Scattered, as if the artist just tossed
them over the oak plank, pansies:
yellow with maroon beard, ruby
edged in pink, plain white, purple
and gold, simple blush, and a few
the hue of wine, periwinkle-lined.
They seem strewn haphazardly
on the torn paper, some upside-down
and overlapping as if the blossom-bag
burst like a mind overrun.

I imagine that Myra Miller, a farmer
of 1,000 acres trained in still life
composition, was not easily overcome.
In her unheated studio, she snipped off
the blossoms, placed each to kiss wood,
and turned them—tiny tea cups—
for balance. The morning of the first
hard frost, her face close to the flowers,
she held her exhale so a word or sigh
slipped from her lips wouldn't moisten
the petals or dull their vibrancy
or send them tumbling over the table,
possibilities of light and line
wrecked with one untensed breath.

Tentative Pregnancy

Lines of chrysalides
quiver in the Butterfly
House and vellums crack
open; delicate wings
emerge glistening, whole.
This hope I pin onto
my body, a bolster for lace-
making, one thousand
bobbins ready for weaving.
Each morning when I wake
to clean sheets, I dismiss
the doubt's pierce: one pin
an arrow launched into
a wobbling, aimless flight.

Ebb & Flow

1.
Hearing the fetal heartbeat
is like putting my ear to a shell;
whispers coalesce into a sound spray.
Then waves: *bump-bump, bump-bump.*
Behind this rhythm, my heart—
an echo, a syncopated splash.

2.
At my feet, the ocean's tidal slap.
I search for scallop, whelk,
conch, clam. My basket fills
until waves fold over a thumb-sized
something, deflated and cold
in my hand. Once, it responded
to touch. Oceans hold with salty
hands. Back and forth it bobs
in a cradle of sand.

3.
I see my fetus floating in amniotic
fluid but hear nothing. Undertow.
Thrown against rocks, I break
into water-carved shells ready
for collection.

Truth Testing

Someone—anyone—please slide
into the sterile room where the chatty doctor
fumbles with the ultra-sound machine, its clanks
and beeps diminishing. Cover my exposed belly
as I stare at the monitor's motionless image,
arms folded under tender breasts. Tell me,
Think of the son you have. Ignore my full-throated
sobs as I whisk tissue after tissue from the box.
When the doctor leaves to "give me time," touch
my shoulder. Reframe this quartet of loss.
Say, *You'll be fine. You'll make the factory
an amusement park.* With long, slow strokes,
caress my hair like a lover might. Predict
I'll understand slight-spoken grief: phrases
exchanged between women when they hug,
hushed confessions lodged in diaries, envelopes
of silent prayer, the glaze crossing a mother's eyes
when she sees big families rough-housing
at the playground. Look me in the eyes.
Whisper, *Someday you'll call them babies.* Tell me.
Tell me! It doesn't matter who you are.
I'll believe.

Plans

At age three, I heard my mom's lessons
for Sunday School, coloring Jesus one idea.
Come Sunday, time ran out. *Later,*
Mom said. *But it was on the plan!* I cried.

When I learned to write, I printed daily menus.
On puppy stationery, I scheduled hours
of leisure: read, write to pen pals, walk dog,
play with baby brother. In high school,
I plotted dreams: college, marriage, house
with garden, career, kids. Check, check, check—
except the last letter of the last one.

Last winter, I graphed my garden in detail.
Stenciled circles intersected. Parallel lines
perfect along blue cells. In summer, zucchini
produced twenty long, green limbs before
too much rain caused root rot. Acorn squash
gave two apple-sized specimens before it
succumbed. I thought of them that September
at my last D&C—fourth miscarriage—
when the doctor scraped to hollow out,
to leave empty and tender.

How perfect plans look on paper, sketched
in colored pencil, penned on glossy calendars.
And still, I yearn to color Jesus, perhaps
in the Parable of the Loaves and Fishes
where he saw hunger and he saw need
and although it wasn't part of the plan,
Jesus created something from nothing;
no, something
                    from love.

When My OB/GYN Said He Didn't Understand Poetry

I worried because my body
is a more complex text.
When he feels the shape
of my uterus, he may not
think pear-shaped yet
an apricot in size, hollow
butternut squash, lightbulb.
He may not consider it a bowl
for a daughter developing inside
with eggs for her daughters,
a set like Grandma's Tupperware
poised to seal away meals,
or nested like Russian dolls,
copies waiting to be twisted off,
revealed. My doctor speaks
the body's language: uterus
tilted toward spine could
mean *incarceration*—womb
snagged on the pelvic bone.
Almond-shaped ovaries pocked
like plum pits—if swollen
with movable lumps—
could be *dermoid*, *endometrioma*,
or *chocolate cysts*. Or nothing
to worry about. He questions
structure, unpuzzles chromosomes,
scrutinizes tensions between
biopsies and blood work, and reads
all this alongside testimony
and history because my flesh,
like a poem, carries mystery:
it produced one child complete

but jettisoned the next four.
My doctor's glossing of my uterine
purse—whether it will fill and stay full
or remain empty—eludes his science.
But when I build a nest of words,
paradox and ambiguity kiss each time,
offspring running down the page.

Swallowing Angels

If summer rains stop being *good*
for crops; if we raise our eyes to clouds,
anxiety's humidity wetting suspense;
if something in us hopes man-made
lakes will choke trees, creeks will lick
the park's swing set, streams will rise
behind homes to run children's glossy balls
away; if, so far, no sewers have backed up;
if no teenager's car has been swept
downriver, then, when five sunny days
pass and the levee starts to ooze
and just before midnight threatens
to breach, we will take stock of danger
that smells of mold, shit, and rotting fish,
and we'll want to stick our fingers
into the gash, into the gush of water
to feel the flood pushing us back, back;
instead, we'll sign up to stack sandbags
and watch water rush over the spillway
like a breaking wave at the beach. Squint
and it'll seem romantic; don't, and it'll look
like dirty water curling over a lip.

Bhoireann, A Stony Place

My five-year-old son and I hop out
of the rental car, tighten our hoods, hold
hands against the wind. On the shale—thin
panes of flagstone, eroded farren—we tiptoe
and peer into grykes to see how far down
cracks open up the earth. By this trip
to Ireland, he's stopped asking for a brother
or sister but coos to strangers' babies bouncing
by in prams. Under a blue sky roughed
with clouds, we tiptoe; plates of slate-colored
rock move under our heels. Between two
limestone sheets, he finds a snail's shell.
Navy blue and ochre, its hues unnatural,
as if someone daubed the coin-sized spiral
with a paintbrush. *No one's home right
now,* he says. *No one will be,* I say, folding
my fingers and slipping it into my pocket.

Design

Recurrent miscarriage: three or more consecutive first trimester miscarriages. Seventy percent of women who have had three miscarriages will carry their next pregnancy to term.

The best seeds germinate at a rate above 65%.

I set concrete block against concrete
    block until the blueprint vanishes
       and a tiny galaxy unfolds
          across my lawn, one finger of God
    curling toward the center. Into this
       chambered nautilus at my garden's
          core, I spread a straw membrane, layer
            blood and bone and soil, shoveling
              with curved hands, skin against fertile earth.

Worms wring their hands in celebration;
      they kiss the sage seeds I've planted, beads
         so light a puff could blow them beyond
           the fence. Miniscule globes, these clusters
of cells. I nudge dill, thyme, cilantro,
      oregano into spring earth like
         a mare nosing her new colt to stand.
            They'll split into root and stem; they'll pulse
              and twitch in darkness like sparks of light.

Inside the sage patch, close to cool dirt,
      my life's design: cotton ball, gauzy
         wrap, cylinder of spun glass. Cocoon.
        Perhaps a butterfly will crack its
    carapace, spread its fine wings. Within
       the sealed sheath, a brown, slender something—
         wisp of silence, twist of DNA,
          a sacred beginning that I can
            cup in my hand's heat, alive or dead.

I'll drizzle golden oil over
           fragrant basil, grind the leaves with cheese,
                pine nuts, and garlic, toss for ribbons
                     of pasta. I'll wrap coins of acorn
           squash with sage leaves, fry them in skillets
                of butter. Needle-spiked rosemary—
                     a stone in the mosaics of meals—
                          I'll snip into minestrone, crush
                               into yams, tuck into sliced roast beef.

In Florida, Ohio, New York,
           blight: a gray-purple dust underneath
                basil. My full oval leaves, pointed
                     at the top like a cat's ear, are free
           so far and a green brighter than jade,
                more verdant than pine. Hue of holly,
                     spring, Ireland, so far from yellow
                          disease and yet easily the wind
                               spreads the spores to start their silent feast.

Only one stalk of feathery dill
           blooms. Twelve velvet tufts—swallowtail
                caterpillars—nestle in fragrant
                     asterisks. Only a centimeter
           long, hair-wide white stripe on black. I pinch
                these pests with thumb and forefinger, pluck
                     all exquisite possibilities
                          save one. I place her on parsley, its
                               abundance easy to sacrifice.

I dream I plant angels on borders
           along wire fences: sweet-smelling
                Angelica archangelica,
                     each seed a bundle of wing and song
           that will sprout and nurture saw-toothed leaves,
                purple-bottomed hollow stems which stretch,
                     lighten to yellow-green. In August,
                          roots push deep into hope, white flowers
                               a canopy, a ceiling of stars.

Thunderstorms press fertile earth into
    sludge: zucchini roots rotted, acorn
        squash stunted at softball size, eggplants
            stillborn in their beds. The sky sloughs off
    cloud-cells. Mosquitoes hatch, spiral up
        from puddles to needle through shirts, jeans.
            I'm tired of tending. And when I
                find a few stalks—for food, for fragrance—
            I can't bring myself to sever them.

Dragonfly-disguised, clarity flits
    over tarragon's slender bookmarks,
        over cilantro curled like newborns'
            hair, over thyme's greening, pear-shaped leaves—
    studs on woody-threaded stems—over
        spears of chives, tender oregano.
            Through its wing—a translucent sphere stretched
            to a teardrop, a miniature
                pane of glass, summer's sunshine refracts.

Cataloguing the Craving

Antidepressant, antioxidant, I'm anything
but anti-you. Chocolate: smooth
as pearls, as patent leather, as the skin
behind an ear. I'll nibble kisses
or cups, haystacks or hearts, fudge
or fondue, bonbons, balls, or barks
for a lift. Organic aphrodisiac.
I dream of Scharffenberger, Cluizel,
Valrhona, Amedei—velvet-wrapped
boxes arriving by post for $100
a pound. For breakfast, I cut devil's
food with cream—American style—
yet I'd lick Mayan bowls of chili-flecked
porridge, sip Aztec cups of froth, savor
the Spaniard's sweeter brew. O bitter
beans! When a craving kicks in, I'll bite
into Mars, Cadbury, Hershey's, or Nestle
but wish for exotic infusions: nutmeg/
pistachio, wasabi/honey, chipotle,
grapefruit, vanilla, violet. I'll settle
down with my beds of gold, peel back
foil one fold at a time, tongue the edge.
Confection prescription. Whether it comes
as truffle, mousse, stick or egg, an ounce
satisfies both the fire and the ache.

Against Melancholy (As Hildegard Defines It)

When black bile settles in me like an army
of buzzing flies, muscles stiffen from my right
shoulder to ear. My eye squints, brow furrows.
Before I realize it, I've inched forward, shifted
in my seat, tilted my hips. The ache lists.
Worse? Exhaustion, as if steel molecules,
subtle in my blood, weigh me down. Lethargic
twilight—my body's ambiguous indigo.

The cause, Hildegard said, is knowing good
but choosing otherwise. Was it my satisfaction
at a loathed-one's bad news? The catch
of judgment at a colleague's words? The friend's
request for help I dismissed as drama?

Hildegard, I want to throw off sorrow
and move bitterness straight on through.
Return me, balanced, to the table.
I'll bandage a nosegay of primrose over
my chest, its heart-shaped petals morphing
into butterflies in my dreams. I'll sleep
with stones of onyx and agate and wake
to cool bruises. I'll sprinkle nutmeg into soup,
oatmeal, coffee. I'll drink quenched wine.
I'll gift jewels to friends, share flowers
with strangers, invite an enemy to tea.
O Inspired One! I'm ready to swim, open-
lipped and kicking, to the surface of my life.

Six Impressions from India Linger

Pushkar was lotus-birthed:
flowers soared through the sky
and landed as buildings;
the calyx, a ring of mountains;
green belly the lands beyond.

The painted elephant stood
still, pink tulips a tiara across
its head. Fleur-de-lis-adorned
ears, cut tusks copper-capped.
His eyes, black coins, blinked.

Turning the corner, I came
face-to-face with a cow: fly-
studded eyes, skin against
corrugated ribs. This sacred
hunger stepped forward.

For food, Kati hennaed
women's bodies. She often
stroked her four-inch scar.
For days, my foot's painting
of curls and loops tingled.

Bracelet of Diana's Tears
linked by silver: each moon-
stone a full cup, swollen seed.
It dangled loose around
my wrist, writing unbound.

The humid breeze smelled
of smoke, wood, and dung
from cooking fires. Monkeys
paced the bathing ghat gates,
beckoning me: *listen, listen.*

The Queen Bee Speaks

Tick, tick, tick zaps
my biological clock—
I've got two years,
so stop messing around
with this cage and queen
candy; inseminate me
already. I see a glint
in your eye, a ruby ring
in your hand. With 1200
eggs dropped daily,
twenty drones just
won't do. I want to spawn
my own hot hive
of workers, a comb
of buzzing bottoms,
a legion of wings
for bee rustlers to round up.
Every day colonies
collapse, but my DNA
will spread from Sacramento
to Bismarck, Houston
to Saratoga Springs.
My progeny will pollinate
almonds, avocado, quince,
coconut, and kiwifruit;
my offspring will defend
their rights to ramondas,
roses, and rhododendrons;
my swarming babies
will fly far and fly high—
and they'll sting this world
to satisfaction.

Visual Thinking Strategies

after *Indian Summer* by Cynthia Reeves

This is my belly's heat
        a New Mexico forest fire
        green organic matter

This is my lover's hand
        on my ass, his tongue
        in my mouth

This is a gourd's ovary, a solar
        flare, the last resort,
        the number five

This means nothing rhymes
        with orange, means a lexicon
        of springs, means Still Life
        with Limes and Grapefruit

This is the moment my lover
        lands on an idea, the second
        his finger settles

This is the skirt of June, a launch
        of mayflies, my spleen's
        dream, fried cumin and chili

This means white-light drips
        water, a child drawing
        on dusty glass, fire as ink

Verge

Where I sit, a pile of storm-struck
twigs can rise in humid columns

of August air, pine needles can glow
in fingers of tree-filtered sunlight,

smoke can seem a halo suspended
in evergreens. Where I reach,

moonlight pools; wind ribbons
around each curved arm. My hair

is a nest of golden filaments. Planks
in this house, my body, creak.

I must float without pruning, wear
fire without burning, thread light

without catching a hand
in the web, build a home in stillness

without splintering arches. I must
breathe to wake up and blaze.

Gladiolus

*In China, this flower serves as heaven's signpost
for the dead.*

When I die, four swords
of blossoms—one for each
of my unborn—will help me
find my way. Their stalks
will be full, green-leaved,
two with supple purple petals—
nearly black—and two pink.
To measure dimensions,
I'll hold their stems
carefully (not too close
to damage) and study
their slopes and curves,
thicknesses and heights.
I'll realize how, close up,
even the pink petals
are touched with gray.
I'll stroke yellow-brushed
throats and the sharp edges
of each leaf. I'll finally
know heaven when I drink
in their scents and discover,
at last, their names.

Epilogue

To My Sixth, Yet Unborn

For you, each day I make a sacrifice:
chores ignored, bitter pills swallowed.
Because, in love, I tossed the rolling dice
there are few luxuries of chance allowed.

We've never met, but I love nonetheless
your fluttering heartbeat and fig-sized flesh.
Because, in love, I gamble on success,
I find my faith in everyone refreshed.

Acknowledgments

Thank you to the editors of the following periodicals and anthologies where these poems first appeared, sometimes with different titles:

Adanna Literary Journal: "How Such Constraints Unbind," "Temporary Innocence," "Tentative Pregnancy," and "Visual Thinking Strategies"
Atlanta Review: "Lessons from India Linger"
The Cape Rock: "Swallowing Angels"
CHEST: American College of Chest Physicians: "Truth Testing"
Cimarron Review: "Bhoireann, A Stony Place"
Cold Mountain Review: "Naming"
Connecticut Review: "Solving for Epilepsy"
Dappled Things: a quarterly of ideas, art, & faith: "Hildegard's Theories Explain My Miscarriage."
Evansville Review: "Pick a Play"
The Fertile Source: "The Learning Curve of Pregnancy Loss" and "When My OB/GYN Said He Didn't Understand Poetry"
Mom Egg Review: "Against Melancholy (As Hildegard Defines It)" and "Permutations of Light"
North Dakota Review: "Epiphany"
Pasque Petals: "When Something Sparks"
Pentimento: Journal of All Things Disability: "Buffaloed"
Rogue Agent: "Boy at Rest"
Shadowbox Magazine: "Portraits Before Epileptic Aphasia"
South Dakota Review: "Framing Loss"

"Verge." *Action, Influence, Voice: Contemporary South Dakota Women.* Eds. Dr. Meredith Redlin, Dr. Christine Stewart-Nuñez, and Dr. Julie Barst. South Dakota Agricultural Heritage Museum, 2015.

"Gladiolus" and "The Queen Bee Speaks." *All We Can Hold: A Collection of Poetry on Motherhood*. Eds: Gregory, Elise and Emily Gwinn. Sage Hill Press, 2016.

Many friends, colleagues, and mentors helped make this book possible. For amazing feedback and encouragement, I thank Dakota Women Poets (Darla Biel, Heidi Czerwiec, Barbara Duffey, Jeanne Emmons, Lindy Obach, Pen Pearson, Marcella Remund, and Normal Wilson), Rochelle Harris and Erika Stevens.

My gratitude to the following institutions for gifts of time and financial support: South Dakota Art Museum (Lynn Verschoor, Lisa Scholten, and Jodi Lundgren), South Dakota State University College of Arts and Sciences (Griffith Grant and Art Fellowship Program), South Dakota State University's Academic and Scholarly Excellence Initiative/Research Support, the South Dakota State University Department of English (especially Jason McEntee and Tiffani Pirner), and the Kimmel Harding Nelson Center for the Arts.

My sincerest thanks to editor/publisher Diane Lockward for believing in this book and selecting it for publication.

Thank you to the medical professionals who cared for me during my multiple miscarriages and two full-term pregnancies, and thank you to the doctors, nurses, psychologists, social workers, technicians, receptionists, and others who help Holden and work hard to solve the mysteries of seizure disorders and the brain.

Thank you to the many artists and scholars whose work informed mine.

Finally, with deep appreciation and love to my family, whose time, energy, and resources help make my amazing life and meaningful work possible.

About the Author

Christine Stewart-Nuñez is the author of three previous books of poetry, *Untrussed* (University of New Mexico Press, 2016), *Keeping Them Alive* (WordTech Editions, 2010), and *Postcard on Parchment* (ABZ Press, 2008) as well as several chapbooks. Her literary work and book reviews have appeared in a variety of magazines, including *Prairie Schooner*, *Calyx*, *Shenandoah*, *Arts & Letters*, and *North American Review*. "An Archeology of Secrets" was a Notable Essay in *Best American Essays 2012* and "Disordered" won the 2014 Lyric Essay Contest at the *Lindenwood Review*. She is a professor in the English Department at South Dakota State University and lives in Brookings, South Dakota, with her husband, architecture professor Brian T. Rex, and her two sons, Holden and Xavier.

CPSIA information can be obtained
at www.ICGtesting.com
Printed in the USA
FSOW02n2042081217
42228FS